CHIA SEED RECIPES

35 Chia Recipes For Better Health, Weight Loss And Longevity

By Katya Johansson

TABLE OF CONTENTS

INTRODUCTION

Chia seeds are the Tesla of superfoods: You've presumably heard a ton about them in some way, yet you don't completely comprehend what the hype is all about.

One ounce of chia seeds contains 11 grams of fiber and 4 grams of protein, with just 129 calories and 9 grams of fat.

They're one of the best plant-based sources of omega-3 unsaturated fats, which can help you lose inches of belly fat. The seeds' rich fiber substance will keep you full for longer and help you fight the urge to snack later in the evenings.

Their one of a kind parity of protein, fats and fiber give you durable vitality.

They retain water, extending to up to 10 times their weight in fluid, helping you feel full and filled. They make for an incredible pre-workout supplement – because as chia seeds are processed, they really discharge water, keeping you hydrated!

It should be clear to you by now why chia seeds are considered to be a superfood.

Let's start cooking some tasty chia seed recipes, shall we?

1. HEALTHY LEMON POPPY SEED LOAF

INGREDIENTS

- 160 g flour
- 12 g preparing powder
- 4 g preparing pop
- 2 g salt
- 170 g coconut oil
- 85 g sugar
- 2 eggs
- 1 yolk
- 170 g yogurt
- 30 g poppy seeds
- 25 g chia seeds
- Pizzazz of 2 lemons
- Vanilla to taste
- 1/2 lemons squeezed (around 70 ml)
- 60 g sugar

METHOD

1. Preheat broiler to 350 degrees F or 175 degrees C.

2. Margarine and flour a piece skillet.

3. Whisk together the flour, heating powder, preparing pop, and salt together. Cream the coconut oil and sugar together until feathery. Gradually include the eggs each one in turn. Include the lemon get-up-and-go, poppy seeds, chia seeds, and vanilla. Beat down the middle the flour, then include the yogurt. Last, include whatever is left of the flour and blend until simply joined. Heat for 45-50 minutes or until a toothpick embedded confesses all.

4. While the piece is heating make the lemon syrup. Heat the lemon squeeze and sugar together until it goes to a stew. When the roll is taken out of the stove, spoon the syrup on top. Leave the chunk in the search for gold hours, or overnight.

2. Amazing Chia Seed Pudding

INGREDIENTS

- For the pudding:
- 2 1/2 glasses unsweetened almond milk
- 1/2 glass Bing fruits, set and split
- 1/2 teaspoon ground cardamom
- 1 teaspoon Sweet Leaf Stevia
- 1 teaspoon vanilla concentrate
- 1/2 container chia seeds
- For the cashew cream:
- 1/4 measure of cashews
- 1/4 container Bing fruits, set and split
- 2 tablespoons chili water
- 1/4 teaspoon vanilla concentrate
- 1/8 teaspoon Sweet Leaf Stevia

METHOD

1. Mix milk, fruits, cardamom, Stevia and vanilla together in a blender on high until smooth. Pour the cherry blend over chia seeds and whisk completely. Let rest for 5

minutes then blend once more. Following 10 minutes, mix once more. Cover and refrigerate no less than 3 hours or overnight.

2. Absorb the cashews water furthermore refrigerate for no less than 3 hours or overnight.

3. To make the cream, mix the fruits in a blender until you have a smooth puree. Deplete and flush the doused cashews and add to the blender alongside icy water. Mix until the cashews are melted, and have a smooth surface. Include vanilla and Stevia and mix until all around joined.

4. Before serving, give the pudding a decent blend and gap into 4 containers; top with cream and more fruits.

3. HEALTHY BANANA CAKE WITH CHIA SEEDS

INGREDIENTS

- 2 mugs almond flour
- ¼ glass tapioca flour
- ¼ glass flaxseed feast
- 1 teaspoon heating pop
- ½ teaspoon salt
- 1 tablespoon chia seeds
- 1 glass bananas, pounded
- 2 eggs, room temperature
- 2 teaspoons vanilla concentrate
- ½ glass coconut milk
- 1/4 glass nectar
- 4 tablespoons coconut oil

METHOD

1. In an expansive dish blend the almond flour, tapioca flour, flaxseed feast, heating pop, salt and chia seeds.

2. In a different dish, cream together coconut oil (not softened) and nectar with a hand blender.

3. Include eggs each one in turn and keep blending.

4. Include crushed banana, vanilla concentrate and coconut milk, blend until completely joined. .

5. Pour wet fixings in with dry fixings and combine with hand blender to frame player.

6. Line 8×8-inch preparing container with material paper, covering two sides. Leave additional long so you have a handle to haul cake out.

7. Pour the blend equally in the container.

8. Prepare at 350°F for 30 minutes or until a toothpick embedded into the middle tells the truth.

9. Set the container on a wire rack while expelling it from the broiler and permit it to cool.

4. Delicious Strawberry Chia Pudding

Ingredients

- 16 ounces crisp strawberries, hulled
- 1/2 glasses (or one 13 1/2-ounce can) coconut milk
- 1/4 glass nectar, or to taste
- 1 vanilla bean, scratched
- 3/4 teaspoon finely ground lime pizzazz
- 1/2 glass chia seeds

Method

1. Place the strawberries, coconut milk, nectar, vanilla, and lime pizzazz in a blender and mix until smooth. Taste and include more nectar if sought.

2. Place the chia seeds in a substantial dish, pour the strawberry blend on top, and whisk altogether. Let stand for 10 minutes and whisk once more.

3. Cover and refrigerate for no less than 4 hours and up to 3 days. Mix the pudding before serving. The more it sits, the thicker the pudding will get to be; on the off chance that you find that it is too thick, speed in a little water (or coconut water, in the event that you have some close by).

4. Spoon into individual glasses or bowls and topping (see proposals beneath).

5. HEALTHY COCONUT CHIA PROTEIN PANCAKES RECIPE

INGREDIENTS

- ¼ container gluten free generally useful flour
- 2 tbsp coconut flour
- 3 tbsp vanilla whey protein powder
- ½ tsp preparing powder
- squeeze of ocean salt
- 1 tbsp chia seeds
- 1 tbsp coconut chips
- 1 egg
- 4 tbsp almond milk

METHOD

1. Consolidate all the dry fixings in a dish. At that point gather wet fixings and mix into a single unit.

2. Heat a dish and coat with coconut oil. Pour 2 tbsp of hitter to frame every flapjack.

3. Cook a couple of minutes. When it begins to rise on top, flip and cook an extra moment or two.

6. WONDERFUL LEMON BISCUITS WITH CHIA SEEDS

INGREDIENTS

For the Muffins

- 2 extensive lemons (yielding ¼ container pizzazz and ⅓ glass juice)
- ½ container sugar
- 1½ mugs generally useful flour
- 1½ teaspoons preparing pop
- ½ teaspoon salt
- 2 teaspoons vanilla
- 2 eggs
- 3 tablespoons oil
- ½ container thick plain Greek yogurt (I didn't utilize low fat)
- ¼ glass drain or cream (I utilized creamer)
- 3 tablespoons chia seeds
- 2 tablespoons poppy seeds
- 2 tablespoons nectar

For the coating

- 1 glass powdered sugar

- 1 tablespoon nectar

- 2 tablespoons drain or cream (I utilized creamer)

- 1 tablespoon salted spread

METHOD

1. Preheat the stove to 375 degrees. Join the lemon pizzazz and the sugar in a medium blending dish. Rub together with your fingers for a couple of minutes to discharge the lemon flavor from the get-up-and-go. Include the flour, heating pop, and salt; blend to join.

2. In a different dish, whisk the lemon juice, vanilla, eggs, oil, yogurt, milk, chia seeds, poppy seeds, and nectar. Add the wet fixings to the dry fixings; mix until simply consolidated.

3. Empty player into lubed biscuit tins; you ought to have the capacity to get 8 vast biscuits. Prepare for 12-14 minutes or until the tops spring back when touched.

4. For the coating, whisk the powdered sugar, nectar, and drain together until smooth. Heat the margarine over medium warmth until liquefied; include the coating blend and mix until gurgling and warm, 1-2 minutes. Expel from warmth and coating biscuits instantly by plunging biscuits topsy turvy into the coating pot or spooning the coating over the tops. Coating ought to set rapidly.

7. HEALTHY APPLE MUG MUFFIN

INGREDIENTS

- Biscuit
- 1 tablespoon grass nourished margarine (or coconut oil)
- 2 tablespoon unsweetened fruit purée (50 grams)
- 1 egg (61 grams)
- 1/4 teaspoon vanilla
- 1 teaspoon maple syrup (10 grams)
- 3 tablespoons almond flour (24 grams) or 2 tablespoons coconut flour
- 1/2 teaspoon cinnamon
- 1/8 teaspoon heating powder (natively constructed)
- Squeeze of salt
- Streusel Topping
- 1 tablespoon apple, finely cleaved
- squeeze of disintegrated walnuts
- squeeze of icy margarine

METHOD

Biscuit (Microwave)

1. Melt the margarine in a microwave safe mug on lower power.

2. Race in the fruit purée, egg, vanilla and maple syrup until very much consolidated

3. Include almond feast, cinnamon, heating powder, and salt and mix for around 30 seconds.

4. Include streusel topping (discretionary) and microwave for 1 minute, 10 seconds

5. Let cool for a couple of minutes and appreciate!

Biscuit (Oven)

1. Preheat stove to 350 Degrees Fahrenheit (176 Celsius)

2. Melt your spread and oil your mug

3. Take after strides 2 and 3 and afterward include your streusel topping (discretionary)

4. Place your mug(s) on a treat sheet and heat for 25 minutes

5. Streusel Topping

6. Join utilizing your fingertips, then sprinkle on top before microwaving.

8. WONDERFUL EGG-FREE APPLE MUG MUFFIN

INGREDIENTS

- 1 tablespoon coconut oil, softened in mug
- 2 tablespoon unsweetened fruit purée
- 1/2 teaspoons ground chia seeds
- 1/2 teaspoons ground flax seeds
- 3 tablespoons water
- 1/4 teaspoon vanilla
- 1 teaspoon maple syrup
- 1/2 teaspoon plain gelatin
- 2 tablespoons coconut flour
- 1 teaspoon arrowroot starch
- 1/2 teaspoon cinnamon
- 1/8 teaspoon preparing powder (custom made)
- Squeeze of salt

METHOD

1. Consolidate and blend your coconut oil, fruit purée, chia seeds, flax seeds, water, vanilla, maple syrup and gelatin in your mug

2. Let sit for 3-5 minutes or more

3. Include your coconut flour, arrowroot, cinnamon, preparing powder and salt, blend well

4. Microwave for 2 1/2 minutes and let cool .Appreciate

8. Tasty Lemon Chia Seed Pancakes with Roasted Strawberries

INGREDIENTS

- For the Roasted Strawberries:
- 1 lb. new strawberries, hulled and cut down the middle
- 1 tablespoon new lemon juice
- 1 tablespoon sugar in the crude
- For the Lemon Chia Seed Pancakes:
- 2 containers white entire wheat flour
- 2 tablespoons granulated sugar
- Get-up-and-go of 2 extensive lemons
- 2 teaspoons preparing powder
- 1 teaspoon preparing pop
- 1/2 teaspoon salt
- 2 containers buttermilk
- 2 huge eggs
- 1/4 container unsalted dissolved spread, cooled
- 1 tablespoon crisp lemon juice
- 1 teaspoon vanilla concentrate
- 1/4 glass chia seeds

- Butter with Canola Oil, for serving

METHOD

1. Preheat the broiler to 375 degrees F. In a medium dish, consolidate the strawberries, lemon squeeze, and sugar. Hurl to join. Pour strawberries on a lubed heating sheet and dish for 20 minutes. Blend the strawberries and meal for an extra 7-10 minutes, until the strawberries are delicate and succulent.

2. While the strawberries are cooking, make the hotcakes. In a little bowl, join the sugar and lemon get-up-and-go. Rub together with your fingers until lemon is fragrant.

3. In a substantial dish, whisk together flour, sugar/lemon blend, heating powder, pop, and salt. In a little bowl, whisk together buttermilk, eggs, liquefied spread, lemon juice, and vanilla. Add wet fixings to the flour blend and mix just until joined. Don't over blend. Tenderly mix in the chia seeds.

4. Heat a frying pan or container to medium low warmth. Coat with cooking splash. Drop around a 1/4 measure of hitter onto warmed skillet. Cook until surface of hotcakes have some air pockets and a couple have blasted, 1 to 2 minutes. Flip precisely with a spatula, and cook until caramelized on the underside, 1 to 2 minutes more. Keep making flapjacks until the hitter is no more. Serve warm with Butter with Canola Oil and simmered strawberries

9. Healthy Honey Chia Dressing for Fruit Salad

Ingredients

- 1 tablespoon crude nectar
- 3 tablespoons lime juice
- 2 tablespoons chia seeds
- 2 mangoes, diced
- 6 strawberries, cut
- 2 kiwifruit, diced
- ½ container blackberries

Method

1. Utilizing a boiling point water shower, warm the nectar somewhat so it is less demanding to mix. Mix in the lime juice and chia seeds.

2. In an expansive dish, join the mangoes, strawberries, kiwifruit, and the blackberries. Blend to blend.

3. Shower the dressing over the natural product serving of mixed greens and hurl delicately to coat. Serve frosty.

10. Delicious Chia Seed Wafer Cookie

INGREDIENTS

- ¾ container chia seeds
- ¼ container whipped spread, relaxed
- 1 egg white
- ½ container coconut sugar
- ½ container agave nectar
- ½ tsp. vanilla concentrate
- ½ container flour
- ¼ tsp. salt
- ¼ tsp. preparing powder

METHOD

1. Formula Directions: Preheat stove to 375 degrees. Place chia seeds on a preparing sheet and toast for 10-15 minutes (ensure they don't smolder).

2. In a huge dish blend coconut sugar, agave, margarine, egg white, vanilla concentrate, flour, and salt, preparing powder and toasted chia seeds together until joined.

3. Utilize a spoon to drop ½-2 tsps. Of batter, around 1 ½ crawls separated onto a heating sheet lined with material

paper. Prepare for 6-8 minutes or until brilliant chestnut.

4. Give treats a chance to cool for around 2 minutes before expelling from heating sheet to a wire rack to cool totally. Store wafers in a water/air proof compartment.

11. Amazing Cauliflower Medallions

Ingredients

- 1/2 head of cauliflower, florets as it were
- 1 expansive egg
- 1 expansive egg white
- 1/2 glass mozzarella
- 1/2 glass onions, diced
- 1/4 glass parsley, hacked
- 3 TBS almond feast
- 2 TBS natural corn feast
- 2 TBS chia seeds
- salt and pepper, to taste
- dried herbs (discretionary)

Method

1. Preheat broiler to 400 degrees F. Oil two treat sheets.

2. Top a pan off with 2 to 3 inches of water, and convey it to bubble. Once the water is bubbled, place the cauliflower florets in the pan. Cook for around 5 minutes. Channel the bubbled water from the pan and run the cauliflower under cool water.

3. Put the cauliflower, cheddar, onions, and parsley in a nourishment processor and blend until everything is finely hacked.

4. Void the cauliflower blend into a dish and mix in the egg and egg white.

5. Include the almond supper, corn dinner, chia seeds, salt, pepper, and any dried herbs, and fold everything into the cauliflower blend.

6. Scoop around a tablespoon of the blend and place it on the treat sheet. Level the blend into little emblems.

7. When all the blend is set on the treat sheets, put the sheets into the broiler.

8. Prepare for around 16 to 20 minutes and flip the emblems part of the way through the heating.

9. Expel the emblems from the stove when they are brilliant chestnut.

12. HEALTHY OVERNIGHT CHOCOLATE CHIA PUDDING

INGREDIENTS

- 1/2 containers (360 ml) Almond Breeze Almond milk Original Unsweetened
- 1/3 container (63 g) chia seeds
- 1/4 container (24 g) cacao or unsweetened cocoa powder
- 2-5 Tbsp (30-75 ml) maple syrup if not mixing (can sub 5-9 dates, set if mixing)
- 1/2 tsp ground cinnamon (discretionary)
- 1/4 tsp ocean salt
- discretionary: 1/2 tsp vanilla concentrate

METHOD

1. Add all fixings with the exception of sweetener to a blending bowl and whisk enthusiastically to consolidate. If not mixing (which I favored!), sweeten to taste with maple syrup right now. On the off chance that mixing, you can sweeten later with maple syrup or dates.

2. Let rest secured in the ice chest overnight or if nothing else 3-5 hours (or until it's accomplished a pudding-like consistency).

3. In the event that mixing, add to a blender and mix until totally smooth and velvety, scratching drawbacks as required. Sweeten to taste.

4. Scraps keep secured in the ice chest for 2-3 days, however best when new.

5. Serve chilled with coveted garnishes, for example, natural product, granola or coconut whipped cream.

13. AMAZING RASPBERRY CHIA SEED JAM

INGREDIENTS

- 1 glass raspberries
- 1 tbsp chia seeds + 2 tbsp water
- 2 tbsp nectar (attempt neighborhood!)

METHOD

1. Absorb chia seeds water for 10 minutes
2. Put all fixings in a blender and heartbeat until joined
3. Store in a glass container in the refrigerator

14. Tasty Lemon Chia Seed Scones

INGREDIENTS

- veggie lover, without gluten, sans dairy
- makes 6 extensive scones
- 2 mugs oat flour (use ensured sans gluten oats if essential)
- 1/2 tsp preparing powder
- 1/2 tsp preparing pop
- 1/4 tsp salt
- 1/4 glass chia seeds
- 1 Tbsp coconut flour
- 1/4 glass coconut oil, solidified in the ice chest
- 1/4 glass nectar (or most loved fluid sweetener, for example, maple syrup)
- 1 egg (1 Tbsp ground flax + 3 Tbsp water for vegetarian egg substitute)
- 1/2 tsp vanilla
- 1 Tbsp lemon juice
- 1 Tbsp lemon pizzazz, or orange get-up-and-go

METHOD

1. Preheat broiler to 350 F and line a heating sheet with material paper. On the off chance that making your own particular oat flour, include two loading measures of antiquated moved oats to the base of a sustenance processor and procedure for 10-15 seconds, or until four-like consistency is come to.

2. Include preparing powder, heating pop, coconut flour, and salt to the oat flour in the nourishment processor. Process 5 seconds. Include the chia seeds and process 3 seconds.

3. Take coconut oil out of the cooler and break separated into little lumps. Add coconut oil pieces to the sustenance processor and procedure 5 seconds. Include egg (of flax-egg), nectar, vanilla, lemon juice, and lemon pizzazz. Process until simply consolidated.

4. Utilizing a spatula, scratch mixture out onto arranged preparing sheet. Let sit around a moment to permit coconut flour to retain a portion of the dampness. Structure batter into a circle, around an inch thick, and cut into six triangles.

5. Prepare for 15 minutes. Take out of the stove and utilizing a sharp blade, isolate the pieces. Prepare another 3-5 minutes to permit the edges to get fresh. Cool on a wire rack.

6. Shower with sweet lemon cashew coat and appreciate

15. Delicious Vanilla-Almond Chia Breakfast Pudding

Ingredients

- 2 containers unsweetened almond milk, custom made or locally acquired
- 1/2 glass chia seeds
- 1/2 teaspoon vanilla concentrate
- 1-2 tablespoons immaculate maple syrup or crude nectar
- Regular natural product for fixing (blueberries, peaches, figs and plums are envisioned here)
- Almonds or different nuts for garnish

Method

1. Join almond milk, chia seeds, vanilla and sweetener in a dish. Blend well until joined and the blend starts to thicken. Store secured in the icebox overnight or for 60 minutes.

2. Blend well before serving and add a touch of water to the pudding on the off chance that it turns out to be too thick. Top with new foods grown from your preferred ground.

16. HEALTHY BANANA-PEANUT BUTTER CHIA SEED MUFFINS

INGREDIENTS

- 1/2 glass Gold Medal™ unbleached generally useful flour
- 1/2 glass Gold Medal™ entire wheat flour
- 3/4 glass ground Nature Valley™ nutty spread crunchy granola bars (around 3 bundles)
- 1/3 glass stuffed light cocoa sugar
- 1 tablespoon heating powder
- 1 glass milk
- 1/2 container smooth nutty spread
- 1 ready huge banana, crushed
- 1 egg
- 2 tablespoons vegetable oil
- 1 teaspoon vanilla
- 1 tablespoon chia seeds

METHOD

1. Heat stove to 350°F. Line a 12-container biscuit tin with paper heating mugs.

2. In a huge dish, whisk together flours, ground granola bars, chestnut sugar and heating powder.

3. In another medium dish, whisk together drain, nutty spread, crushed banana, egg, vegetable oil and vanilla until smooth.

4. Include wet fixings and chia seeds to dry fixings. Blend until simply consolidated.

5. Separate hitter among paper heating containers. Heat biscuits until a toothpick embedded in the middle confesses all, around 20-25 minutes. Expel from broiler. Expel biscuits from biscuit tin and cool on a cooling rack.

17. HEALTHY CHIA OATMEAL BREAKFAST COOKIES

INGREDIENTS

- 1½ Tablespoons chia seeds
- ¼ container Almond Breeze unsweetened vanilla almond milk
- 2 ready bananas, crushed
- ¾ container antiquated oats
- ¼ container unsweetened destroyed coconut
- ¼ container hacked dates
- ¼ container dull chocolate lumps or carob chips
- 1 Tablespoon smooth almond spread
- extensive squeeze of cinnamon

METHOD

1. Preheat stove to 350°.

2. In a little bowl, blend together the chia seeds and almond drain and let the blend sit for around 10 minutes, or until the chia seeds have made a pleasant gel-like consistency.

3. Empty the chia seed gel into a medium measured blending bowl and include the crushed bananas, oats,

coconut, almond margarine and cinnamon until all around joined.

4. Delicately blend in the dates and chocolate lumps.

5. Scoop out mixture (around 1-2 tablespoons worth) onto a heating stone or a lubed treat sheet and utilize a fork to press the batter down a little to make to a greater extent a treat shape. You ought to get around 15 treats.

6. Place in broiler and heat for 17-20 minutes, or until the base of the treats have cooked a minor piece.

7. Take them out, let cool and appreciate.

18. BEST GLUTEN-FREE CHIA TORTILLAS

INGREDIENTS

- 1/2 glass chia seeds
- 1/3 glass crude buckwheat groats
- 1/2 container ground flax seed
- 1/4 container sorghum flour
- 2 containers warm water
- 1 teaspoon salt
- 2 tablespoons olive oil

METHOD

1. Preheat the stove to 350F. Line 2 heating sheets with material paper. Cut 2 additional bits of material paper the same size as the container.

2. Place the chia seeds in a dry, rapid blender. Mix to pound into a fine flour. Fill a dish and rush in the warm water gradually. Give the blend a chance to sit while you set up the remaining fixings, close to 3 minutes.

3. Place the crude buckwheat groats in the blender and drudgery into a fine flour. Include the buckwheat flour, flax, sorghum, salt, and olive oil to the dish and blend enthusiastically to join. The hitter will be thick and sticky.

4. Scoop 1/3 measure of the hitter onto the lined treat sheet. You ought to have the capacity to fit 2 tortillas for each dish so space another 1/3 measure of hitter on the same preparing sheet. Place the additional bit of material paper on the player and press in a roundabout movement to spread the tortilla. They ought to be around 1/4 crawl thick, making them too thin will make them break.

5. Prepare the tortillas for 6-7 minutes on one side. Flip and back for an expansion 3-4 minutes. The material paper ought to peel effectively off the tortillas when they are finished.

6. When you expel them from the broiler permit them to chill 1 minute before taking the paper. Try not to let the tortillas completely cool inside the parchment or they will stick. Place the tortillas on a cooling rack. Rehash with the remaining hitter. Appreciate!

7. Store the remains with bits of parchment or wax paper in-between them in a fixed pack in the fridge.

8. Makes 7-9 wraps.

19. TASTY BLUEBERRY TOASTED COCONUT PARFAITS WITH PISTACHIOS

INGREDIENTS

- 6 Tbsp chia seeds
- 2 containers almond or soy milk, vanilla or plain
- 2 Tbsp grade B maple syrup, coconut syrup or agave syrup
- Reduce sweetener by one tablespoon if your non-dairy milk is on the sweet side.
- squeeze of salt
- 1/8 tsp vanilla concentrate
- 1/4 tsp cinnamon
- 1/2 glass blueberries (overlay or mix in)
- toasted coconut:
- 4 Tbsp unsweetened coconut
- topping:
- 1/4 glass crisp blueberries
- 3 tsp crude pistachios

METHOD

- Around 6+ hours before serving parfaits, set up the chia pudding. You can just energetically mix all fixings together or do my low speed blender strategy. I include the milk, vanilla, sweetener, salt and cinnamon - turn blender on to least speed. Gradually pour in chia seeds so they don't adhere to the sides of the blender. Mix on low for around 2-3 minutes to kick off the chia seed plumping procedure. Blueberries: you can either overlay in the 1/2 measure of blueberries or mix them directly into the pudding.

- Exchange your chia blend to a little bowl or extensive jug. Cover and place int he ice chest for no less than six hours. Around thirty minutes and one hour subsequent to setting in the cooler I get a kick out of the chance to give my pudding a couple blends to twirl the chia seeds a bit. This keeps them from clustering up at the base or top of the glass. This progression is choices, you can simply do an energetic blend just before serving as well.

- At the point when prepared to plan parfaits, finely slash your pistachios and put aside. For the coconut, warm the coconut in a dry skillet over high warmth. Warm just until the edges begin to cocoa and "toast." Set aside.

- Add chia pudding to tall parfait glasses. You can mix a few or the greater part of the coconut directly into the pudding or simply layer it on top of the pudding in the parfait glass. Top with the new blueberries, more toasted coconut and pistachios. I want to serve my chia pudding with a mammoth side dish of additional blueberries, since you can never have excessively numerous blueberries on the table.

20. HEALTHY CORNMEAL AND CHIA SEED CRUSTED TILAPIA

INGREDIENTS

- 4 boneless tilapia filets (1 pound absolute), tapped dry
- A couple dashes of Kosher salt and ground dark pepper
- 1.5 Tablespoons low-fat mayonnaise
- 3/4 container cornmeal
- 1/2 teaspoon chia seeds*
- 1/2 teaspoon garlic powder
- olive oil cooking splash

METHOD

1. Preheat the stove to 400 degrees Fahrenheit.

2. On a plate, hurl together the cornmeal, chia seeds, garlic powder, and a dash each of salt and pepper.

3. Place a cooking rack onto a preparing sheet, splash delicately with olive oil/non-stick cooking shower and put aside.

4. Sprinkle some salt and pepper onto every bit of fish, trailed by a smear a portion of the mayonnaise and afterward upset the fish into the cornmeal blend. Press

immovably and afterward flip the fish over and place onto the cooking rack.

5. Heat for 15-20 minutes relying upon the thickness of the fish.

21. Amazing Cinnamon with Ginger and Chia Seeds

INGREDIENTS

- 1 medium ready plantain (7oz or 200g once peeled)
- 1 glass pumpkin (8oz)
- 2 tablespoons chia seeds
- 1/2 teaspoon heating pop
- 1 teaspoon heating powder
- 1/4 teaspoon cinnamon
- 1/8 teaspoon cloves
- 1/4 teaspoon ground ginger
- 1/4 teaspoon nutmeg
- 1/4 glass coconut sugar (1/4oz)
- 2 tablespoons coconut oil (1oz), fluid

METHOD

1. Pre-heat broiler to 350 degrees.
2. Put every single dry fixing into a dish, whisk the fixings.

3. Next peel your plantain and puree in a sustenance processor or blender.

4. Once pureed include into dry fixings dish.

5. Mix till all joined.

6. Include pumpkin puree and coconut oil.

7. Hitter will be somewhat thick.

8. Get your container and scoop your hitter into every opening. On the other hand into your 8 inch skillet.

9. I daintily oiled my container with coconut oil.

10. Prepare for around 20 minutes or till toothpick confesses all

22. WONDERFUL CHIA SEED CRACKERS

INGREDIENTS

- Makes 3-4 dozen little/medium wafers (I made 48 little saltines)
- 1 huge unfenced natural egg
- 2 tablespoons chia seeds
- 1 container/3.8 oz/110 gr almond dinner/flour
- 6 tablespoons ground Parmesan cheddar
- ½ teaspoon fine grain ocean salt
- ¼ teaspoon ground dark pepper
- ¼ teaspoon ground cayenne pepper (discretionary)

METHOD

1. In a huge dish consolidate all fixings and blend until a mixture ball shapes.

2. On the off chance that the mixture is excessively wet and doesn't shape into a ball include further almond dinner, one tablespoon at once. Then again, if the mixture is excessively dry include some water ½ teaspoon at once.

3. Wrap mixture in waxed paper or plastic wrap, and refrigerate for no less than 30 minutes, and up to 3 days.

4. Expel the mixture from the cooler 10 minutes before you are good to go it out.

5. Preheat the broiler to 325°F (160°C) and line two preparing sheets with material paper.

6. Place mixture between two sheets of material paper, press into a level plate, and move it with a moving pin until the batter is 1/8-crawl thick. Cut into fancied shapes utilizing a blade or cutter. Any remaining mixture can be rerolled for more saltines.

7. With a spatula, exchange the wafers to the readied heating sheets, permitting about an inch between saltines.

8. Prepare until the bottoms are cooked, and the tops interpretation of a decent measure of shading too - 12 to 15 minutes, contingent upon how thick your saltines really are. Check the stove regularly to counteract smoldering the saltines (I've taken in the most difficult way possible!)

9. Turn the sheets part of the way through preparing (or when the saltines in the back appear as though they are searing more rapidly than the front).

10. Permit to cool before putting away.

23. DELICIOUS CHIA MEATBALLS

INGREDIENTS

- 1 lb. grass-nourished ground meat (prescribed no leaner than 85%)
- 2 T. natural tomato glue
- 2 cloves garlic, minced
- 2 t. herbs de Provence
- 1 t. ocean salt
- 1 t. ground pepper
- 2 T. chia seeds
- 2 t. 100% Pure Avocado Oil, for sauteing

METHOD

1. Join all fixings aside from the avocado oil in an expansive bowl and blend well with a fork. Let rest for 5-10 minutes so the chia can do its thing.

2. Heat a huge skillet over medium warmth and include the avocado oil. Scoop 8 balls and pat into a round shape. Cook meatballs until chestnut, turning on no less than 3 sides. Move meatballs to a plate to rest (they won't be completely cooked yet will get done with cooking later in the sauce) and deplete everything except 1-2 T. of oil from the skillet.

24. Amazing Spicy Pineapple Pepper Chia Seed Jam

Ingredients

- 2 Cups Peeled, Cored, Chopped, Pineapple
- ¼ Cup Diced Red Pepper
- ¼ Teaspoon (or More) Red Pepper Flakes
- 2 Tablespoons Honey
- 2-3 Cups Water
- Tablespoons Chia Seeds (Black or White)

Method

1. Join the pineapple, pepper, pepper chips, nectar and some the water in a medium-sized nonstick pan. Convey the blend to a tender bubble over medium warmth.

2. When bubbling, diminish the warmth to medium-low, and keep on cooking for an extra 30 minutes, until the fluid has totally dissipated and the pineapple is delicate. Include water as vital, in light of how succulent your pineapple is to begin with. Basically, the pineapple ought to be separated, and the fixings ought to seem as though they are gelling.

3. Discretionary: At this point,I like to give the entire skillet (off the warmth) a snappy shot with my submersion blender. On the off chance that you don't have a submersion blender, you can rapidly beat ½ of the blend in a normal blender or a nourishment processor. This progression is totally up to you, and ward upon the consistency you need to accomplish, yet I lean toward my "jam" to be on the smoother side. Once mixed, empty the blend over into your skillet.

4. Add the chia seeds to the blend, and mix continually (the seeds will adhere to the skillet), for roughly five minutes. Expel from the warmth.

5. Permit to cool, as the "jam" will keep on solidifying as the temperature diminishes.

25. Delicious Honey Almond Chia Granola

Ingredients

- 2 containers moved oats
- 3/4 containers crude almonds, generally hacked
- 1/2 container chia seeds
- 1/2 container destroyed unsweetened coconut
- 1/3 container nectar (I utilized crude, unfiltered)
- 1/3 container coconut oil
- 1 tablespoon coconut sugar (or chestnut sugar)
- 1/2 teaspoon salt
- 1 teaspoon vanilla concentrate
- 2 tablespoons egg white (from one egg)
- Makes around 24 ounces
-

Method

1. Preheat the broiler to 300°F and line a heating sheet with material paper.
2. In a vast dish, join moved oats, almonds, chia seeds, salt and destroyed coconut.

3. In a different little bowl, join the nectar, coconut oil, coconut sugar, vanilla concentrate and two tablespoons of egg white.

4. Empty wet fixings into the dry and mix until everything is blended altogether.

5. Spread blend onto preparing sheet so it is a substantial, level rectangular shape.

6. Prepare in stove for around 45 minutes or until brilliant chestnut.

7. On the off chance that you lean toward not to have substantial lumps of granola then expel it from the stove at 30 minutes and mix before cooking the rest of the time. Something else, permit granola to cool for no less than thirty minutes before separating into extensive lumps.

8. Store in an impermeable compartment for up to two weeks or main a parfait with crisply cut peaches and expend promptly

26. DELICIOUS CHOCOLATE AND GINGER CHIA SEED COOKIES

INGREDIENTS

- 1 tablespoon chia seeds
- 3 tablespoons almond milk
- 1 container moved oats (gluten free on the off chance that you are gluten delicate)
- 1/2 teaspoon preparing pop
- 1/4 teaspoon preparing powder
- 1/8 teaspoon salt
- 1/4 container regular unadulterated sweetener
- 1 tablespoon newly ground ginger
- 1/2 teaspoon vanilla concentrate
- 1 tablespoons maple syrup
- 4 tablespoons coconut oil at room temperature
- 75g dull chocolate, cleaved or chips
- 2 tablespoons sweetened ginger, meagerly slashed

METHOD

1. Preheat the stove to 350 F/175 C

2. Consolidate the chia seeds and the almond milk in a little bowl and put aside for no less than 10 minutes

3. Mix the oats in a nourishment processor until you have a coarse flour. Include the preparing pop, heating powder, sugar and salt and heartbeat just to blend. Next include the ginger, vanilla, maple syrup, coconut oil and chia seed blend and heartbeat until the mixture frames a ball. Expel from the sustenance processor and spot between two sheets of material paper so you can undoubtedly move it out without staying (you could likewise put the mixture in the ice chest wrapped firmly in plastic wrap up to 24 hours). Roll the batter with a moving pin until you have a rectangular shape around 1/2 inch think. Utilizing a treat cutter or the edge of a glass, cut out circles or whatever other shape and place on a material lined heating sheet

4. Heat in the stove for around 18-20 minutes until the treats have puffed up a bit in center and are somewhat chestnut on top

5. Expel from the broiler and let cool on a rack

6. Once the treats have cooled totally, dissolve the chocolate in a twofold kettle over stewing water. Be mindful so as not to give the base of the pot a chance to touch the water or the chocolate won't soften pleasantly, and blend frequently. On the other hand, you could dissolve the chocolate in the microwave at 20 second interims, blending admirably in the middle.

7. Plunge the cooled treats in the liquefied chocolate, about midway, and brighten with a couple pieced of sugar coated ginger

8. Give the chocolate a chance to solidify (you can speed this up by setting in the cooler) and store the treats in an

impermeable holder or keep them in the cooler until they are prepared to be delighted in!

27. Tasty Chocolate Chia Pudding

INGREDIENTS

- 2 1/2 glasses coconut milk
- 1/4 glass Dutch prepared cocoa powder
- 1/4 glass rice malt syrup
- 1/2 glass chia seeds
- 2 glasses blended solidified berries

METHOD

1. Place coconut milk in an expansive blending dish, sifter over coconut powder and mix well to consolidate. Include rice malt syrup, blend well to join, then include chia seeds and mix well for around 5 minutes until pudding starts to thicken as the chia seeds broaden.

2. Partition blend between serving glasses or containers, spread in stick wrap. Place in refrigerator for 4 hours or overnight.

3. Place solidified berries in a pan with some water and place on low warmth, twirling dish at times until berries are just defrosted. Put aside until prepared to serve.

4. To serve, top puddings with berries and squeeze.

28. Delicious Cranberry and Chia Seed Coconut Scones

Ingredients

- 150g coconut oil
- 2 tablespoons nectar
- 1 container whole meal flour
- 1/2 teaspoon bicarbonate pop
- 1 container moved oats
- 1/2 container coconut palm sugar (see Note)
- 1/2 container parched coconut
- 1/2 container dried cranberries, slashed
- 1/2 container coarsely slashed pistachios
- 1/3 container dark chia seeds

Method

1. Preheat stove to 180°C or 160°C fan-power. Line 2 vast preparing plate with heating paper. Place coconut oil and nectar in a little pan over medium-low warmth. Cook, blending, for 2 to 3 minutes or until consolidated and smooth. Expel from warmth. Permit to cool.

2. Filter flour and bicarbonate of pop into an extensive dish. Include husks from strainer. Blend in oats, sugar, coconut, cranberries, and pistachio and chia seeds. Include cooled coconut oil blend and mix until very much consolidated (the blend will even now brittle).

3. Put solidly pressed level 1/4 container measures of blend on arranged plate, permitting 2cm for spreading. Level marginally and reshape, squeezing with fingertips, until a 10cm wide circle. Prepare for 15 minutes or until brilliant. Permit to cool totally on plate.

29. HEALTHY WHEAT CHIA SEED PANCAKES

INGREDIENTS

- Makes 8–10 flapjacks
- 1 c. entire wheat flour
- 1/2 c. antiquated oats
- 1 c. milk
- 1 egg
- 1 tbsp. canola oil
- 2 tbsp. nectar
- 1/2 tsp. pumpkin pie flavor
- 1/2 tsp. preparing powder
- 1/4 tsp. salt
- 1 tbsp. chia seeds (in addition to additional for embellishment)
- Syrup or other craved fixings

METHOD

1. Splash frying pan or container with cooking shower and warmth to a medium warmth. Beat egg and include drain and oil. In a different dish, consolidate flour, oats,

pumpkin pie zest, preparing powder and salt. Abating mix flour blend into egg blend.

2. Include nectar and mix until combined At the latest possible time, mix in chia seeds. Pour 1/4 c. bits of player onto iron and cook until edges of hotcakes begin to air pocket and bottoms are light chestnut. Flip and cook until focuses are totally done (around three to four minutes). Top with syrup, extra chia seeds or fancied fixings and appreciate.

30. AMAZING RAW HEMP CHIA SEED BARS

INGREDIENTS

DRY INGREDIENTS

- 3 1/2 glasses natural speedy moved oats (without gluten, if necessary)
- 1/2 glass natural hemp seeds
- 1/2 glass natural chia seeds
- 1/4 glass natural flaxseeds (newly ground)
- 3/4 glasses natural almonds (newly ground in small pieces)

WET INGREDIENTS

- 1/2 container natural crude nectar (or other fluid sweetener for vegetarian)
- 1/2 container natural fruit purée
- 3/4 containers natural almond margarine
- 1/2 container natural coconut oil (softened/fluid)
- 1/2 teaspoon natural vanilla concentrate

METHOD

1. Placed flaxseeds into an espresso processor and drudgery into a powder. Put aside.

2. Placed almonds into a nourishment processor and procedure until they are in minor pieces. Put aside.

3. In an extensive dish, combine every single dry fixing (oats, hemp seeds, chia seeds, ground flax seeds, ground almonds and coconut, if utilized).

4. In a medium estimated dish, combine every wet fixing (crude nectar or other fluid sweetener, fruit purée, almond margarine, softened coconut oil and vanilla concentrate).

5. Take the wet fixing blend and join in the expansive dish with the dry fixings and mix until all around consolidated, utilizing your hands if necessary.

6. Put the blend in a 8 x 8 glass heating dish and press the blend solidly.

7. Put in the fridge or cooler to chill or until the blend is firm.

8. Cut into even size bars or littler measured squares.

31. Healthy Cornmeal and Chia Seed Crusted Tilapia

Ingredients

- 4 boneless tilapia filets (1 pound all out), tapped dry
- A couple dashes of Kosher salt and ground dark pepper
- 1.5 Tablespoons low-fat mayonnaise
- 3/4 glass cornmeal
- 1/2 teaspoon chia seeds*
- 1/2 teaspoon garlic powder
- olive oil cooking shower

Method

1. Preheat the stove to 400 degrees Fahrenheit.
2. On a plate, hurl together the cornmeal, chia seeds, garlic powder, and a dash each of salt and pepper.
3. Place a cooking rack onto a heating sheet, splash gently with olive oil/non-stick cooking shower and put aside.
4. Sprinkle some salt and pepper onto every bit of fish, trailed by a smear a portion of the mayonnaise and after that rearrange the fish into the cornmeal blend. Press

solidly and afterward flip the fish over and place onto the cooking rack.

5. Prepare for 15-20 minutes relying upon the thickness of the fish

32. Tasty Raspberry Coconut Chia Pudding Pops

INGREDIENTS

- 1/2 container lite coconut milk
- 1/2 container unsweetened almond milk
- 3/4 container raspberries
- 2 tbsp chia seeds
- 1 tbsp sweetened destroyed coconut
- 8 drops Nu-Naturals fluid stevia (or sugar/nectar to taste)

METHOD

1. Consolidate all fixings in an extensive holder. Blend well and close compartment; refrigerate 4 hours so the chia extends.
2. Fill 4 popsicle shape and stop overnight.

33. Delicious Avocado Fruit Salad with Chia Yogurt Dressing

INGREDIENTS

- 1 grapefruit
- 1 pear
- 1 orange
- 1 avocado
- 1 mango
- 10 strawberries
- 1/2 lemon, juice crushed
- 1/4 glass 0% Greek yogurt
- 2 tbsp immaculate vanilla concentrate
- 1/4 glass chia seeds

METHOD

1. Wash, peel, core and remove seeds (if vital) and cut into fancied size pieces organic products. Add to a dish.

2. To make the dressing, in a different dish whisk together Greek yogurt, lemon juice, vanilla concentrate and chia seeds. Pour over the foods grown from the ground sufficiently only to consolidate. Serve chilled.

3. Store secured in the fridge for up to 1 day. Mix delicately before serving to lift the juices from the base of the dish.

34. HEALTHY MINT CHOCOLATE CHIA SEED PUDDING

INGREDIENTS

- 1/3 glass sugar
- 1/3 glass water
- 1 modest bunch entire mint clears out
- 1/3 glass entire chia seeds
- 2 tablespoon cocoa powder
- 1/2 teaspoon vanilla concentrate
- squeeze of ocean salt
- 1 glass unsweetened almond milk

METHOD

1. In a little pot, combine sugar, water and mint clears out

2. Heat to the point of boiling and expel from warming, permitting to cool before utilizing (it will thicken as it cools)

3. Expel mint leaves from syrup before utilizing

4. In a fast blender or dish, combine chia seeds, cocoa powder, vanilla concentrate, ocean salt, almond milk and two tablespoons of cooled mint straightforward syrup (you will have additional — pour it on dessert or all the more new strawberries!)

5. Separate blend into two 8-ounce artisan bumps and refrigerate for no less than two hours before serving

6. Serve chilled

35. HEALTHY BLUEBERRY CHIA BLAST SMOOTHIE

INGREDIENTS

- 1 and 1/2 mugs coconut milk refreshment (I utilized So Delicious brand here)
- 1/2 container delicate luxurious tofu
- 1 tablespoon nectar
- 2 tablespoons chia seeds
- 1 scoop (around 1-2 tablespoons) vanilla whey protein powder
- 1 container solidified blueberries

METHOD

Consolidate the greater part of the fixings in a blender and mix until smooth. Serve instantly.